HIGH
TRIGLYCERIDES
COOKBOOK & FOOD LIST

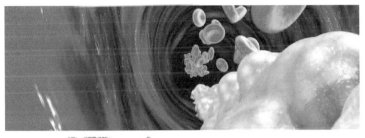

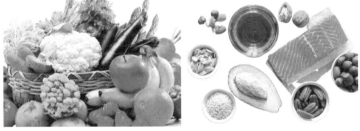

A Diet Cookbook with Quick And Simple Healthy Recipes To Lower Triglycerides _ 21-Day Meal Plan and Food List Included: Lose Weight, Improve Heart Health, and Boost Energy by Lowering Your Triglycerir'

MARY CALIN

Contents

INTRODUCTION.. 4

CHAPTER ONE 7

What are triglycerides? 7

Why are high triglycerides a problem? 7

What are the symptoms of high triglycerides?....... 8

How are high triglycerides diagnosed?.................. 9

What are the treatment options for high
triglycerides? 9

How to lower your triglycerides with a diet 10

CHAPTER TWO 13

FOODS TO EAT 13

FOODS TO AVOID 34

CHAPTER THREE... 37

TRIGLYCERIDE LOWERING MEAL PLAN 37

WEEK 1 38

Week 2 40

Week 3 41

CHAPTER FOUR 43

TRIGLYCERIDE LOWERING BREAKFAST
RECIPES 43

CHAPTER FIVE 65

TRIGLYCERIDE-LOWERING LUNCH RECIPES
.... 65

CHAPTER SIX 85

TRIGLYCERIDE-LOWERING DINNER RECIPES
.... 85

CHAPTER SEVEN 105

TRIGLYCERIDE-LOWERING SNACKS RECIPES
.... 105

Conclusion 117

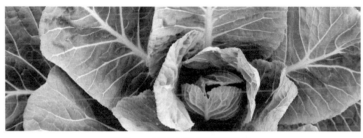

LEAFY GREENS

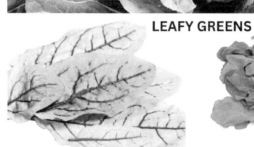

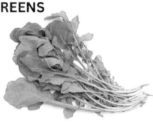

INTRODUCTION

Are you tired of feeling sluggish and unhealthy?

Do you have high triglycerides?

Are you feeling that way? You're not the only one. Triglycerides are a type of fat that can make you more likely to get heart disease, stroke, and other health problems. Millions of people around the world have high levels of them.

No worries, though! Eating differently can help lower your fats and make you healthier. Adding more heart-healthy foods like fruits, veggies, and whole grains into your meals can help lower triglyceride levels. Beyond that, doing regular exercise and keeping a healthy weight can also help improve your health and lower your risk of health problems.

This cookbook has all the information you need to follow a high triglyceride diet. If you want to lower your triglycerides and improve your health in general, this book will teach you everything you need to know.

Not only does this book give you detailed information on the right foods to eat, but it also gives you useful tips and tasty recipes to make these changes easy to make in your daily life. You can control your triglyceride levels and live a healthier, more balanced life by following the tips and rules in this complete guide.

Imagine a life where you feel energetic, healthy, and in control of your health.

Imagine a life where you're not at risk of heart disease, stroke, or other serious health problems.

That life is possible with a high triglyceride diet.

CHAPTER ONE

What are triglycerides?

Triglycerides are a form of fat that is found in the blood. They are the most common type of fat found in your body's fat cells. When you eat, your body turns any calories that aren't immediately used into triglycerides. Triglycerides are then stored in fat cells for future use. Triglycerides provide energy to the body in between meals. When your body requires energy, it releases triglycerides from your fat cells into your bloodstream. The triglycerides are subsequently broken down by your liver into fatty acids, which your body utilizes for energy.

Why are high triglycerides a problem?

Triglyceride levels that are too high can make you more likely to get heart disease, stroke, and other health issues. Triglycerides that are too high can cause fat to build up in your vessels.

This can make your arteries stiffer and smaller, leading to atherosclerosis (plaque building up in the vessels). Atherosclerosis can make you more likely to have a heart attack, stroke, or other heart issue.

Also, having high triglycerides can make you more likely to get pancreatitis, which is a very bad disease of the pancreas.

What are the symptoms of high triglycerides?

Most people with high triglycerides do not have any symptoms. However, some people may have the following symptoms:

- Fatty deposits under the skin (xanthomas)
- Enlarged liver
- Spleen enlargement
- Milky white appearance of the blood (lipaemia)

How are high triglycerides diagnosed?

High triglycerides are diagnosed with a blood test called a lipid panel. A lipid panel measures the levels of different types of fat in your blood, including triglycerides.

What are the treatment options for high triglycerides?

The main treatment for high triglycerides is lifestyle changes, such as:

- Losing weight if you are overweight or obese
- Eating a healthy diet
- Exercising regularly
- Quitting smoking
- Limiting alcohol intake

If lifestyle changes are not enough to lower your triglycerides, your doctor may prescribe medication.

How to lower your triglycerides with a diet

Here are some tips for lowering your triglycerides with diet:

- Lots of fruits and veggies are good for you. Plant-based foods are high in fiber and low in fat and calories. They also have a lot of minerals and vitamins, which are good for your health.

- When you can, choose whole grains over processed grains. There is a lot of fiber in whole grains, which can help drop cholesterol and triglycerides.

- Lean protein sources like beans, fish, and chicken are good choices. Avoid foods that are high in fat, like beef, bacon, and sausage.

- Cut back on trans and heavy fats. High triglyceride levels can be caused by saturated and trans fats. Foods that are high in saturated fats include fatty foods, full-fat dairy, and tropical oils. Processed foods, like fried foods, margarine, and baked goods, contain trans fats.

- Cut down on sweet drinks. Some drinks that are high in sugar and calories are soda, juice, and sports drinks. They can make cholesterol levels go up and make you gain weight.

- Drink less booze. Trolleybilides can go up when you drink alcohol. Limiting or not drinking booze at all is important if you have high triglycerides.

CHAPTER TWO

FOODS TO EAT

FOOD GROUP	FOODS TO EAT
Fruits	All fruits, except for coconuts
Vegetables	All vegetables, except for starchy vegetables such as potatoes, corn, and peas
Whole grains	Oats, brown rice, quinoa, whole-wheat bread and pasta
Lean protein	Fish, chicken, beans, lentils, tofu
Healthy fats	Avocados, nuts, seeds, olive oil
Other	Low-fat dairy products, unsweetened beverages

FRUIT GROUP

Fruit	Nutritional Information (per serving)	Why to Eat
Apple	95 calories, 25 grams (g) carbohydrates, 4 g fiber, 14 mg vitamin C	Apples are a good source of fiber and vitamin C. Fiber can help lower your triglycerides and cholesterol levels. Vitamin C is an antioxidant that can help protect your cells from damage.
Banana	105 calories, 27 g carbohydrates, 3 g fiber, 422 mg potassium	Bananas are a good source of potassium and vitamin B6. Potassium can help lower your blood pressure. Vitamin B6 is essential for energy metabolism.
Berries	50-80 calories per cup, 10-15 g carbohydrates per cup, 3-5 g fiber per cup, 15-25 mg vitamin C per cup	Berries are a good source of antioxidants and fiber. Antioxidants can help protect your cells from damage. Fiber can help lower your triglycerides and cholesterol levels.

Citrus fruits	50-80 calories per cup, 10-15 g carbohydrates per cup, 2-4 g fiber per cup, 30-50 mg vitamin C per cup	Citrus fruits are a good source of vitamin C and folate. Vitamin C is an antioxidant that can help protect your cells from damage. Folate is important for cell growth and repair.
Melons	50-80 calories per cup, 10-15 g carbohydrates per cup, 2-4 g fiber per cup, 20-40 mg vitamin C per cup	Melons are a good source of vitamins A and C. Vitamin A is important for vision and immune function. Vitamin C is an antioxidant that can help protect your cells from damage.
Pears	100 calories, 25 g carbohydrates, 6 g fiber, 10 mg vitamin C	Pears are a good source of fiber and potassium. Fiber can help lower your triglycerides and cholesterol levels. Potassium can help lower your blood pressure.

VEGETABLE GROUP

Vegetable	Nutritional Information (per serving)	Why to Eat
Broccoli	31 calories, 6 g carbohydrates, 3 g fiber, 100 mg vitamin C, 89 mg vitamin K	Broccoli is a good source of fiber, vitamins C and K, and potassium. Fiber can help lower your triglycerides and cholesterol levels. Vitamins C and K are essential for blood clotting and bone health.
Brussels sprouts	35 calories, 8 g carbohydrates, 4 g fiber, 89 mg vitamin C, 114 mg vitamin K	Brussels sprouts are a good source of fiber, vitamins C and K, and folate. Fiber can help lower your triglycerides and cholesterol levels. Vitamins C and K are essential for blood clotting and bone health. Folate is important for cell growth and repair.

Cabbage	22 calories, 5 g carbohydrates, 2 g fiber, 37 mg vitamin C, 72 mg vitamin K	Cabbage is a good source of fiber, vitamins C and K, and potassium. Fiber can help lower your triglycerides and cholesterol levels. Vitamins C and K are essential for blood clotting and bone health.
Cauliflower	25 calories, 5 g carbohydrates, 3 g fiber, 53 mg vitamin C, 77 mg vitamin K	Cauliflower is a good source of fiber, vitamins C and K, and folate. Fiber can help lower your triglycerides and cholesterol levels. Vitamins C and K are essential for blood clotting and bone health. Folate is important for cell growth and repair.

Carrots	25 calories, 6 g carbohydrates, 2 g fiber, 736 IU vitamin A, 12 mg vitamin C	Carrots are a good source of fiber, vitamins A and C, and potassium. Fiber can help lower your triglycerides and cholesterol levels. Vitamin A is important for vision and immune function. Vitamin C is an antioxidant that can help protect your cells from damage.
Celery	16 calories, 4 g carbohydrates, 1 g fiber, 14 mg vitamin K	Celery is a good source of fiber and vitamin K. Fiber can help lower your triglycerides and cholesterol levels. Vitamin K is essential for blood clotting and bone health.
Cucumbers	16 calories, 4 g carbohydrates, 1 g fiber, 11 mg vitamin K	Cucumbers are a good source of water and fiber. Fiber can help lower your triglycerides and cholesterol levels.

Eggplant	25 calories, 6 g carbohydrates, 3 g fiber, 11 mg vitamin K	Eggplant is a good source of fiber and potassium. Fiber can help lower your triglycerides and cholesterol levels. Potassium can help lower your blood pressure.
Leafy greens	5-10 calories per cup, 1-2 g carbohydrates per cup, 1-2 g fiber per cup, 10-20 mg vitamin C per cup, 100-200 mg vitamin K per cup	Leafy greens are a good source of fiber, vitamins C and K, and folate. Fiber can help lower your triglycerides and cholesterol levels. Vitamins C and K are essential for blood clotting and bone health. Folate is important for cell growth and repair.
Mushrooms	15 calories, 3 g carbohydrates, 2 g fiber, 2 mg vitamin B2, 10 mg vitamin D	Mushrooms are a good source of fiber, vitamins B2 and D, and potassium. Fiber can help lower your triglycerides and cholesterol levels. Vitamins B2 and D are essential for energy metabolism and bone health.

Onions	40 calories, 10 g carbohydrates, 2 g fiber, 12 mg vitamin C, 4 mg vitamin B6	Onions are a good source of fiber, vitamins C and B6, and potassium. Fiber can help lower your triglycerides and cholesterol levels. Vitamins C and B6 are essential for energy metabolism and immune function.
Peppers	25 calories, 6 g carbohydrates, 2 g fiber, 95 mg vitamin C, 10 mg vitamin A	Peppers are a good source of fiber, vitamins C and A, and potassium. Fiber can help lower your triglycerides and cholesterol levels. Vitamins C and A are essential for energy metabolism and immune function.
Tomatoes	25 calories, 6 g carbohydrates, 1 g fiber, 12 mg vitamin C, 760 IU vitamin A	Tomatoes are a good source of fiber, vitamins C and A, and potassium. Fiber can help lower your triglycerides and cholesterol levels. Vitamins C and A are essential for energy metabolism and immune function.

WHOLE GRAINS GROUP

Whole Grain	Nutritional Information (per serving)	Why to Eat
Oats	150 calories, 30 g carbohydrates, 4 g fiber, 5 g protein	Oats are a good source of fiber, beta-glucans, and protein. Fiber can help lower your triglycerides and cholesterol levels. Beta-glucans are a type of soluble fiber that can help reduce the absorption of cholesterol. Protein is essential for building and repairing muscle tissue.
Brown rice	216 calories, 48 g carbohydrates, 3 g fiber, 5 g protein	Brown rice is a good source of fiber and manganese. Fiber can help lower your triglycerides and cholesterol levels. Manganese is an essential mineral for bone health and metabolism.
Quinoa	222 calories, 40 g carbohydrates, 8 g fiber, 8 g protein	Quinoa is a good source of fiber, protein, and iron. Fiber can help lower your triglycerides and cholesterol levels. Protein is essential for building and repairing muscle tissue. Iron is essential for oxygen transport.

Whole-wheat bread	160 calories, 34 g carbohydrates, 4 g fiber, 7 g protein	Whole-wheat bread is a good source of fiber, complex carbohydrates, and B vitamins. Fiber can help lower your triglycerides and cholesterol levels. Complex carbohydrates provide a steady source of energy. B vitamins are essential for energy metabolism and brain function.
Whole-wheat pasta	220 calories, 45 g carbohydrates, 7 g fiber, 13 g protein	Whole-wheat pasta is a good source of fiber, complex carbohydrates, and B vitamins. Fiber can help lower your triglycerides and cholesterol levels. Complex carbohydrates provide a steady source of energy. B vitamins are essential for energy metabolism and brain function.

LEAN PROTEIN

Lean Protein	Nutritional Information (per serving)	Why to Eat
Salmon	206 calories, 30 g protein, 4 g fat, 2 g omega-3 fatty acids	Salmon is a good source of protein, omega-3 fatty acids, and vitamin D. Protein is essential for building and repairing muscle tissue. Omega-3 fatty acids can help lower triglycerides and improve cholesterol levels. Vitamin D is important for bone health and immune function.
Chicken breast	165 calories, 31 g protein, 3 g fat	Chicken breast is a good source of protein and niacin. Protein is essential for building and repairing muscle tissue. Niacin is essential for energy metabolism and skin health.
Beans	240 calories, 15 g protein, 13 g fiber	Beans are a good source of protein, fiber, and folate. Protein is essential for building and repairing muscle tissue. Fiber can help lower triglycerides and cholesterol levels. Folate is important for cell growth and repair.

Lentils	230 calories, 18 g protein, 13 g fiber	Lentils are a good source of protein, fiber, and folate. Protein is essential for building and repairing muscle tissue. Fiber can help lower triglycerides and cholesterol levels. Folate is important for cell growth and repair.
Tofu	70 calories, 8 g protein, 5 g fat	Tofu is a good source of protein, iron, and calcium. Protein is essential for building and repairing muscle tissue. Iron is essential for oxygen transport. Calcium is important for bone health.

HEALTHY FATS GROUP

Healthy Fat	Nutritional Information (per serving)	Why to Eat
Avocados	240 calories, 20 g fat (13 g monounsaturated fat, 2 g polyunsaturated fat, 5 g saturated fat), 4 g fiber	Avocados are a good source of monounsaturated fats, fiber, and potassium. Monounsaturated fats can help lower triglycerides and LDL cholesterol levels. Fiber can help lower triglycerides and cholesterol levels. Potassium can help lower blood pressure.
Nuts	160-200 calories per serving, 6-10 g fat (mostly monounsaturated and polyunsaturated fats), 2-4 g fiber, 3-5 g protein	Nuts are a good source of monounsaturated and polyunsaturated fats, fiber, and protein. Monounsaturated and polyunsaturated fats can help lower triglycerides and LDL cholesterol levels. Fiber can help lower triglycerides and cholesterol levels. Protein is essential for building and repairing muscle tissue.

Seeds	160-200 calories per serving, 6-10 g fat (mostly monounsaturated and polyunsaturated fats), 3-5 g fiber, 3-5 g protein	Seeds are a good source of monounsaturated and polyunsaturated fats, fiber, and protein. Monounsaturated and polyunsaturated fats can help lower triglycerides and LDL cholesterol levels. Fiber can help lower triglycerides and cholesterol levels. Protein is essential for building and repairing muscle tissue.
Olive oil	120 calories per tablespoon, 14 g fat (9 g monounsaturated fat, 2 g polyunsaturated fat, 1 g saturated fat)	Olive oil is a good source of monounsaturated fat. Monounsaturated fat can help lower triglycerides and LDL cholesterol levels.

OTHER GROUP

Food	Nutritional Information (per serving)	Why to Eat
Low-fat dairy products	100-150 calories per serving, 8-12 g protein, 5-8 g fat, 300-400 mg calcium	Low-fat dairy products are a good source of protein, calcium, and vitamin D. Protein is essential for building and repairing muscle tissue. Calcium is important for bone health. Vitamin D is important for bone health and immune function.
Unsweetened beverages	0-10 calories per serving, 0 g fat, 0 g sugar	Unsweetened beverages are a good way to stay hydrated without adding calories or sugar to your diet.

Low-fat dairy products include:

- Skim milk
- 1% milk
- 2% milk
- Low-fat yogurt
- Low-fat cheese, such as mozzarella, cheddar, and Swiss
- Fat-free cottage cheese
- Fat-free ricotta cheese

Low-fat dairy products are a good source of protein, calcium, and vitamin D. Protein is essential for building and repairing muscle tissue. Calcium is important for bone health. Vitamin D is important for bone health and immune function.

Here are some tips for choosing low-fat dairy products:

- Look for products that say "low-fat" or "fat-free" on the label.
- Compare the fat content of different products to choose the one that is lowest in fat.
- Choose plain yogurt over flavored yogurt, as flavored yogurt often contains added sugar.

- Choose low-fat cheese over regular cheese, as low-fat cheese is lower in saturated fat and calories.

- Use cottage cheese or ricotta cheese instead of cream cheese in recipes.

You can include low-fat dairy products in your diet in a variety of ways. For example, you can add skim milk to your coffee or cereal, eat low-fat yogurt for breakfast or lunch, or use low-fat cheese in sandwiches or casseroles.

Unsweetened beverages include:

- Water
- Unsweetened tea
- Unsweetened coffee
- Club soda
- Sparkling water
- Sugar-free beverages, such as diet soda and seltzer water

Unsweetened beverages are a good way to stay hydrated without adding calories or sugar to your diet. Sugar can contribute to weight gain, high triglycerides, and other health problems.

Here are some tips for choosing unsweetened beverages:

- Avoid sugary drinks, such as soda, juice, and sports drinks.

- Choose unsweetened tea and coffee over sweetened versions.

- Add flavor to your water with lemon or lime juice, cucumber slices, or mint leaves.

- Choose sparkling water instead of regular soda.

- If you choose to drink sugar-free beverages, make sure to read the label carefully to make sure that they do not contain any artificial sweeteners that you may be sensitive to.

You can include unsweetened beverages in your diet in a variety of ways. For example, you can drink water throughout the day, have a cup of unsweetened tea or coffee in the morning, or enjoy a sparkling water with your meal.

It is important to note that even unsweetened beverages can contain caffeine. Caffeine can cause side effects such as anxiety, insomnia, and headaches. If you are sensitive to caffeine, it is important to limit your intake of unsweetened tea, coffee, and other caffeinated beverages.

NUTS AND SEEDS INCLUDES	
Nuts:	Seeds
Almonds	Chia seed
Brazil nuts	Flaxseed
Cashews	Hemp seeds
Hazelnuts	Pumpkin seeds
Macadamia nuts	Sesame seeds
Peanuts	Sunflower seeds
Pecans	
Pistachios	
Walnuts	

TIPS FOR CHOOSING AND STORING NUTS AND SEEDS:

- Choose unsalted or lightly salted nuts and seeds.
- Avoid nuts and seeds that are roasted in oil.
- Store nuts and seeds in an airtight container in a cool, dark place.

Nuts and seeds can be a healthy and delicious part of your diet. Just be sure to eat them in moderation, as they are high in calories.

List of leafy greens:

1. Arugula
2. Beet greens
3. Bok choy
4. Collard greens
5. Dandelion greens
6. Kale
7. Mustard greens
8. Romaine lettuce
9. Spinach
10. Swiss chard
11. Turnip greens
12. Watercress

Leafy greens can be eaten raw, cooked, or juiced. They can be added to salads, sandwiches, wraps, and stir-fries. Leafy greens can also be used to make smoothies and soups.

Here are some tips for incorporating leafy greens into your diet:

- Add a handful of leafy greens to your morning smoothie.
- Top your sandwich or wrap with leafy greens.
- Sauté leafy greens with garlic and olive oil for a quick and easy side dish.
- Add leafy greens to soups and stews.
- Juice leafy greens for a nutritious beverage.

Leafy greens are a delicious and nutritious way to improve your overall health.

FOODS TO AVOID

Food Group	Foods to Avoid	Why to Avoid
Saturated and trans fats	Fatty meats, butter, full-fat dairy products, fried foods, processed foods	Saturated and trans fats can raise triglycerides.
Refined grains	White bread, white rice, pasta, sugary cereals	Refined grains are quickly broken down into sugar in the body, which can raise triglycerides.
Sugary drinks	Soda, juice, sports drinks, sweetened coffee and tea	Sugary drinks are high in calories and can contribute to weight gain, which can raise triglycerides.
Alcohol	Alcohol can raise triglycerides.	

Tips for avoiding foods that can raise triglycerides:

- Read food labels carefully and choose foods that are low in saturated and trans fats, sugar, and sodium.

- Limit your intake of processed foods.

- Choose lean meats and low-fat dairy products.

- Eat plenty of fruits and vegetables.

- Choose whole grains over refined grains.

- Drink water instead of sugary drinks.

- Limit your intake of alcohol.

CHAPTER THREE

TRIGLYCERIDE LOWERING MEAL PLAN

WEEK 1

Day	Breakfast	Snack	Lunch	Dinner
1	Oatmeal with berries and nuts	Yogurt parfait with fruit and granola	Salad with grilled chicken or fish	Salmon with roasted vegetables
2	Whole-wheat toast with avocado and eggs	Hard-boiled eggs	Soup and sandwich on whole-wheat bread	Chicken stir-fry with brown rice
3	Smoothie made with fruits, vegetables, and yogurt	Nuts and seeds	Lentil soup	Lentil tacos
4	Chia pudding with berries and nuts	Hard-boiled eggs and whole-wheat crackers	Tuna salad sandwich on whole-wheat bread	Leftovers from dinner

5	Tofu scramble with vegetables	Fruits and vegetables	Quinoa salad with vegetables and chickpeas	Turkey sandwich on whole-wheat bread with avocado and vegetables
6	Whole-wheat pancakes with fruit and yogurt	Yogurt	Black bean burgers with sweet potato fries	Spaghetti with whole-wheat pasta and tomato sauce
7	Hard-boiled eggs and whole-wheat crackers	Fruits and vegetables	Grilled chicken breast with brown rice and vegetables	Grilled salmon with roasted vegetables

Week 2

Day	Breakfast	Snack	Lunch	Dinner
1	Yogurt parfait with fruit and granola	Hard-boiled eggs	Lentil soup	Tofu tacos with quinoa and vegetables
2	Smoothie made with fruits, vegetables, and yogurt	Nuts and seeds	Soup and sandwich on whole wheat bread	Black bean burgers with sweet potato fries
3	Whole-wheat toast with avocado and eggs	Hard-boiled eggs and whole-wheat crackers	Salad with grilled chicken or fish	Spaghetti with whole-wheat pasta and tomato sauce
4	Chia pudding with berries and nuts	Fruits and vegetables	Quinoa salad with vegetables and chickpeas	Turkey sandwich on whole-wheat bread with avocado and vegetables
5	Tofu scramble with vegetables	Yogurt	Leftovers from dinner	Grilled chicken breast with brown rice and vegetables
6	Whole-wheat pancakes with fruit and yogurt	Hard-boiled eggs	Lentil soup	Grilled salmon with roasted vegetables
7	Hard-boiled eggs and whole-wheat crackers	Fruits and vegetables	Tuna salad sandwich on whole-wheat bread	Lentil tacos

Week 3

Day	Breakfast	Snack	Lunch	Dinner
1	Smoothie made with fruits, vegetables, and yogurt	Nuts and seeds	Soup and sandwich on whole-wheat bread	Black bean burgers with sweet potato fries
2	Whole-wheat toast with avocado and eggs	Hard-boiled eggs and whole-wheat crackers	Salad with grilled chicken or fish	Spaghetti with whole-wheat pasta and tomato sauce
3	Chia pudding with berries and nuts	Fruits and vegetables	Quinoa salad with vegetables and chickpeas	Turkey sandwich on whole-wheat bread with avocado and vegetables
4	Tofu scramble with vegetables	Yogurt	Leftovers from dinner	Grilled chicken breast with brown rice and vegetables

5	Whole-wheat pancakes with fruit and yogurt	Hard-boiled eggs	Lentil soup	Grilled salmon with roasted vegetables
6	Hard-boiled eggs and whole-wheat crackers	Fruits and vegetables	Tuna salad sandwich on whole-wheat bread	Lentil tacos
7	Smoothie made with fruits, vegetables, and yogurt	Nuts and seeds	Soup and sandwich on whole-wheat bread	Black bean burgers with sweet potato fries

CHAPTER FOUR

TRIGLYCERIDE LOWERING

BREAKFAST RECIPES

Oatmeal with berries and nuts

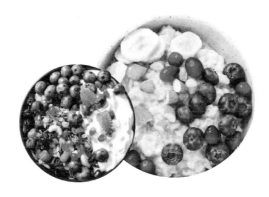

Prep time: 5 minutes

If you want a healthy and tasty breakfast that is also high in fiber and nutrients, try oatmeal. On top of that, it has a lot of protein, which can help you feel full. Adding nuts and berries to your oatmeal is a great way to make it taste better and make it healthier.

Nutritional information:

One serving of oatmeal with berries and nuts contains approximately:

- Calories: 250   Fat: 5 grams
- Carbohydrates: 40 grams
- Fiber: 10 grams Protein: 10 grams

Cooking Steps	Ingredients

1. In a small pot, mix the oats with the milk or water. On high heat, bring to a boil. Low-level the heat and let it cook for 5 minutes, or until the oats are fully cooked.
2. Take the pan off the heat and add the nuts, berries, and cinnamon, if using. Add honey or maple syrup to taste to make it sweeter.
3. Serve right away and enjoy!

- 1/2 cup rolled oats
- 1 cup water or milk
- 1/4 cup berries
- 1 tablespoon nuts
- 1/2 teaspoon ground cinnamon (optional)
- Honey or maple syrup to taste (optional)

Yogurt parfait with fruit and granola

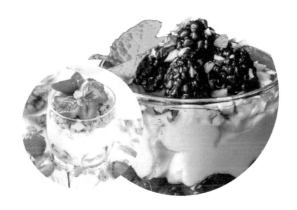

Prep time: 5 minutes

Making a yogurt spread for breakfast is quick and easy, and it tastes great too. Also, they're a great way to use up yogurt and veggies that you have left over.

Nutritional information:

One serving of yogurt parfait with fruit and granola contains approximately:

- Calories: 250
- Fat: 5 grams
- Carbohydrates: 40 grams
- Fiber: 10 grams
- Protein: 10 grams

Cooking Steps	Ingredients
1. Put the cereal, fruit, and yogurt in a jar or glass in a certain order. 2. Do this again and again until the jar or glass is full. 3. Serve right away and enjoy!	- 1 cup plain yogurt - 1/2 cup fruit (such as berries, sliced banana, or chopped apple) - 1/4 cup granola

Whole-wheat toast with avocado and eggs

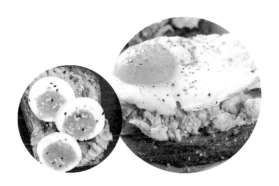

Prep time: 5 minutes

A filling and healthy breakfast is whole-wheat toast with avocado and eggs. It has a lot of fiber, protein, and good fats.

Nutritional information:

One serving of whole-wheat toast with avocado and eggs contains approximately:

- Calories: 250
- Fat: 10 grams
- Carbohydrates: 30 grams
- Fiber: 5 grams
- Protein: 15 grams

Cooking Steps	Ingredients
1. Toast up the whole-wheat bread.	- 1 slice whole-wheat bread
2. Use a fork to spread the avocado on the toast.	- 1/4 avocado, mashed
3. How you like it, cook the egg.	- 1 egg
4. On top of the avocado toast, put the egg.	- Salt and pepper to taste
5. Add pepper and salt to taste.	
6. Serve right away and enjoy!	

Smoothie made with fruits, vegetables, and yogurt

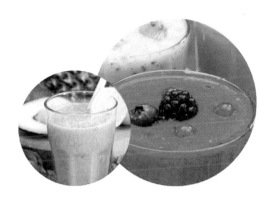

Prep time: 5 minutes

Smoothies are a great way to eat enough veggies and fruits every day. They're also a quick and tasty way to start the day.

Nutritional information:

One serving of smoothie made with fruits, vegetables, and yogurt contains approximately:

- Calories: 250
- Fat: 5 grams
- Carbohydrates: 40 grams
- Fiber: 10 grams
- Protein: 10 grams

Cooking Steps	Ingredients
1. Putting everything in a blender and blending it until it's smooth. 2. Serve right away and enjoy!	- 1 cup yogurt - 1/2 cup fruit (such as berries, banana, or mango) - 1/2 cup vegetables (such as spinach, kale, or cucumber) - 1/2 cup water or milk

Chia Pudding with Berries and Nuts

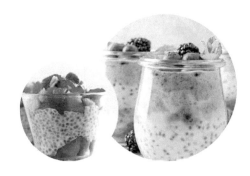

Prep time: 5 minutes (plus overnight chilling time)

If you want a healthy and tasty breakfast that is also full of nutrients, try chia pudding. Besides that, it has a lot of fiber and protein, which can help you feel full. Adding nuts and berries to your chia pudding is a great way to make it taste better and make it healthier.

Nutritional information:

One serving of chia pudding with berries and nuts contains approximately:

- Calories: 250
- Fat: 10 grams
- Carbohydrates: 30 grams
- Fiber: 10 grams
- Protein: 10 grams

Cooking Steps	Ingredients
1. In a bowl or jar, mix the chia seeds with the milk of your choice. Use a stir to mix. 2. Put the jar or bowl in the fridge overnight with the top lid. 3. Stir the chia pudding again in the morning. 4. Place the nuts, berries, and cinnamon on top. 5. Add honey or maple syrup to taste to make it sweeter. 6. Serve right away and enjoy!	- 1/2 cup chia seeds - 1 cup milk of your choice (such as almond milk, oat milk, or cow's milk) - 1/4 cup berries - 1 tablespoon nuts - 1/2 teaspoon ground cinnamon (optional) - Honey or maple syrup to taste (optional)

Hard-Boiled Eggs with Whole-Wheat Toast and Fruit

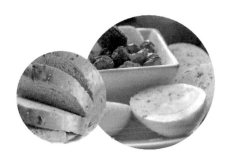

Prep time: 5 minutes

Hard-boiled eggs are a quick and healthy way to start the day. They have a lot of protein and good fats. Toast made from whole wheat has a lot of fiber and complicated carbs. A lot of vitamins, minerals, and enzymes can be found in fruit.

Nutritional information:

One serving of hard-boiled eggs with whole-wheat toast and fruit contains approximately:

- Calories: 250
- Fat: 10 grams
- Carbohydrates: 30 grams
- Fiber: 5 grams, Protein: 15 grams

Cooking Steps	Ingredients
1. Cut the hard-boiled eggs in half lengthwise.	- 2 hard-boiled eggs
2. Toast up the whole-wheat bread.	- 1 slice whole-wheat toast
3. Put the eggs that have been hard-boiled on the toast.	- 1/2 cup fruit (such as berries, banana, or sliced apple)
4. Add any fruit you like on top.	
5. Serve right away and enjoy!	

Breakfast Burrito Made with Whole-Wheat Tortilla, Eggs, Vegetables, and Salsa

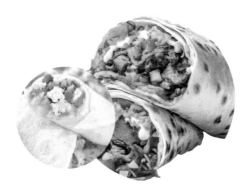

Prep time: 5 minutes

Breakfast burritos are a filling and tasty way to start the day. You can get a lot of protein, fiber, and complex carbs from them. You can also make them your own by adding different toppings and veggies.

Nutritional information:

One serving of a breakfast burrito made with a whole-wheat tortilla, eggs, vegetables, and salsa contains approximately: Calories: 250

- Fat: 10 grams
- Carbohydrates: 30 grams
- Fiber: 5 grams, Protein: 15 grams

Cooking Steps	Ingredients
1. You can use the oven or a skillet to warm up the whole-wheat tortilla. 2. The egg should be spread out on the bread. 3. Choose your veggies and salsa to go with it. 4. Wrap the tortilla up and serve right away.	- 1 whole-wheat tortilla - 1 egg, scrambled - 1/4 cup vegetables (such as spinach, kale, or bell peppers) - 1 tablespoon salsa

Vegetable Omelet with Whole-Wheat Toast

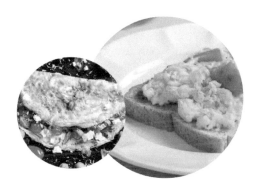

Prep time: 5 minutes

Omelets with vegetables are a tasty and healthy way to start the day. You can get a lot of protein and veggies from them. Toast made from whole wheat has a lot of fiber and complicated carbs.

Nutritional information:

One serving of a vegetable omelet with whole-wheat toast contains approximately: Calories: 250

- Fat: 10 grams
- Carbohydrates: 30 grams
- Fiber: 5 grams
- Protein: 15 grams

Cooking Steps	Ingredients
1. In a bowl, mix the egg, veggies, salt, and pepper using a whisk. 2. Set the small pan on medium heat. 3. Butter or oil should be added in small amounts to the pan. 4. Put the egg mix into the pan and cook for two to three minutes on each side, or until the eggs are fully cooked. 5. Serve the egg on whole-wheat toast after folding it in half.	- 1 egg - 1/4 cup vegetables (such as spinach, kale, or bell peppers), chopped - 1/4 teaspoon salt - 1/4 teaspoon pepper - 1 slice whole-wheat toast

Tofu Scramble with Vegetables

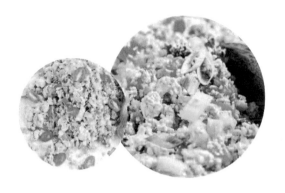

Prep time: 5 minutes

Tofu scramble is a veggie and healthy way to start the day. Protein and veggies can be found in it in good amounts.

Nutritional information:

One serving of tofu scramble with vegetables contains approximately:

- Calories: 200
- Fat: 10 grams
- Carbohydrates: 20 grams
- Fiber: 5 grams
- Protein: 15 grams

Cooking Steps	Ingredients
1. Set the small pan on medium heat.	- 1/2 block tofu, crumbled
2. Butter or oil should be added in small amounts to the pan.	- 1/4 cup vegetables (such as spinach, kale,
3. Put the veggies and tofu in the pan. Cook for two to three minutes, or until the vegetables get soft.	or bell peppers), chopped
	- 1/4 teaspoon salt
	- 1/4 teaspoon pepper
4. Add pepper and salt to taste.	
5. Serve right away.	

Whole-wheat pancakes with Fruit and Yogurt

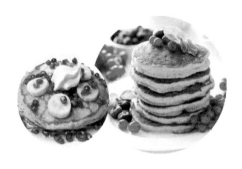

Prep time: 10 minutes

Whole-wheat pancakes are a tasty and healthy way to start the day. These foods have a lot of fiber and complicated carbs. Adding fruit and yogurt to pancakes is a great way to make them taste better and make them healthier.

Nutritional information:

One serving of whole-wheat pancakes with fruit and yogurt contains approximately: Calories: 300

- Fat: 10 grams
- Carbohydrates: 40 grams
- Fiber: 5 grams
- Protein: 10 grams

Cooking Steps	Ingredients
1. In a large mixing basin, combine the flour, baking powder, baking soda, and salt.	- 1 cup whole-wheat flour - 1 teaspoon baking powder
2. Whisk together the milk, egg, and vegetable oil in a separate basin.	- 1/4 teaspoon baking soda
3. Whisk together the wet and dry ingredients until just mixed.	- 1/4 teaspoon salt - 1 cup milk of your choice
4. Melt butter in a large skillet over medium heat.	- 1 egg
5. To the skillet, add a tiny amount of butter or oil.	- 1 tablespoon vegetable oil
6. For each pancake, pour 1/4 cup batter into the skillet.	- 1/4 cup fruit (such as berries, banana, or sliced apple)
7. Cook for approximately 2-3 minutes per side, or until golden brown.	- 1/4 cup yogurt
8. Serve with your favorite fruit and yogurt.	

CHAPTER FIVE

TRIGLYCERIDE-LOWERING

LUNCH RECIPES

Salad with Grilled Chicken or Fish

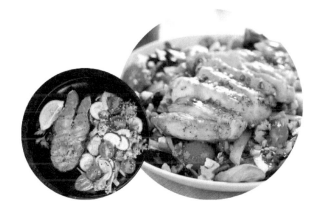

Prep time: 10 minutes

Salads are a delicious way to obtain your daily serving of fruits and vegetables. They are also low in fat and calories. Adding grilled chicken or fish to your salad increases its protein value and makes it more filling.

Nutritional information:

One serving of salad with grilled chicken or fish contains approximately:

- Calories: 250

- Fat: 5 grams

- Carbohydrates: 30 grams

- Protein: 20 grams

Cooking Steps	Ingredients
1. In a mixing bowl, combine the mixed greens, grilled chicken or fish, veggies, and dressing. 2. To mix, toss everything together. 3. Serve right away.	- 2 cups mixed greens - 1/2 cup grilled chicken or fish, chopped - 1/4 cup vegetables (such as tomatoes, cucumbers, or carrots), chopped - 2 tablespoons dressing of your choice

Soup and Sandwich on Whole-Wheat Bread

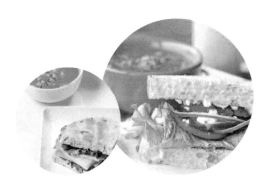

Prep time: 5 minutes

A healthy and convenient lunch option is soup and a sandwich on whole-wheat bread. Soup is an excellent method to obtain your daily serving of vegetables and water. Whole-wheat bread is high in fiber and complex carbs.

Nutritional information:

One serving of soup and a sandwich on whole-wheat bread contains approximately: Calories: 300

- Fat: 10 grams
- Carbohydrates: 40 grams
- Fiber: 5 grams
- Protein: 20 grams

Cooking Steps	Ingredients
1. Cook the soup according to the package instructions. 2. With your sandwich, enjoy the soup.	- 1 cup soup of your choice - 1 sandwich on whole-wheat bread with lean protein and vegetables (such as a turkey sandwich on whole-wheat bread with lettuce and tomato)

Lentil Soup

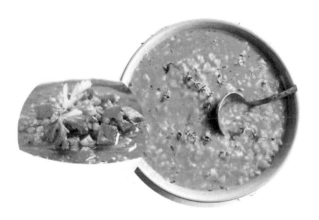

Prep time: 15 minutes _ Cook time: 30 minutes

Lentil soup is a healthy and delicious lunch option. It is a good source of protein, fiber, and complex carbohydrates. It is also low in calories and fat.

Nutritional information:

One serving of lentil soup contains approximately:

- Calories: 200
- Fat: 5 grams
- Carbohydrates: 30 grams
- Fiber: 10 grams
- Protein: 15 grams

Cooking Steps	Ingredients
1. In a large pot, combine all of the ingredients. 2. Bring to a boil, then reduce to low heat and continue to cook for 30 minutes, or until the lentils are cooked.. 3. Serve immediately.	- 1 cup lentils - 2 cups vegetable broth - 1/2 cup chopped onion - 1/2 cup chopped carrots - 1/4 cup chopped celery - 1/4 teaspoon garlic powder - 1/4 teaspoon black pepper

Tuna Salad Sandwich on Whole-Wheat Bread

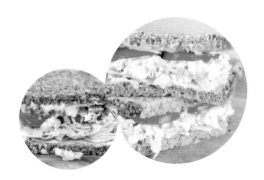

Prep time: 5 minutes

A tuna salad sandwich on whole-wheat bread is a nutritious and convenient lunch option. The tuna salad is rich in protein and omega-3 fatty acids. Whole-wheat bread is rich in complex carbohydrates and dietary fiber.

Nutritional information:

One serving of a tuna salad sandwich on whole-wheat bread contains approximately:

- Calories: 250   Fat: 10 grams
- Carbohydrates: 30 grams
- Fiber: 5 grams
- Protein: 20 grams

Cooking Steps	Ingredients
1. Combine the tuna, mayonnaise, celery, onion, salt, and pepper in a bowl. 2. Spread the tuna salad on the slices of whole-wheat bread. 3. Enjoy!	- 1 can tuna, drained - 1/4 cup mayonnaise - 1/4 cup chopped celery - 1 tablespoon chopped onion - 1/4 teaspoon salt - 1/4 teaspoon black pepper - 2 slices whole-wheat bread

Quinoa Salad with Vegetables and Chickpeas

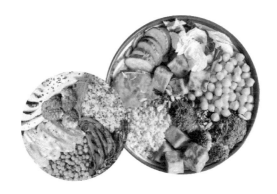

Prep time: 10 minutes

Quinoa is a nutritious and adaptable grain that is high in protein, fiber, and complex carbs. It also has a minimal calorie and fat content. Adding vegetables and chickpeas to your quinoa salad boosts its nutritional content and makes it more filling.

Nutritional information:

One serving of quinoa salad with vegetables and chickpeas contains approximately: Calories: 250

- Fat: 5 grams

- Carbohydrates: 30 grams

- Fiber: 10 grams

- Protein: 15 grams

Cooking Steps	Ingredients
1. In a mixing bowl, combine the quinoa, veggies, chickpeas, olive oil, lemon juice, salt, and pepper. 2. To mix, toss everything together. 3. Serve right away.	- 1 cup quinoa, cooked - 1/2 cup vegetables (such as tomatoes, cucumbers, or carrots), chopped - 1/4 cup chickpeas, drained and rinsed - 1 tablespoon olive oil - 1 tablespoon lemon juice - 1/4 teaspoon salt - 1/4 teaspoon black pepper

Tofu Sandwich on Whole-Wheat Bread

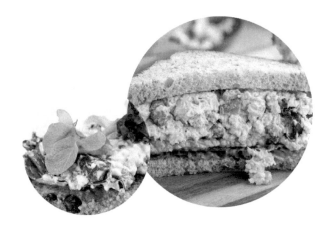

Prep time: 5 minutes

A tofu sandwich on whole-wheat bread is a nutritious and tasty lunch choice. Tofu is high in both protein and calcium. Whole-wheat bread is high in fiber and complex carbs.

Nutritional information:

One serving of a tofu sandwich on whole-wheat bread contains approximately: Calories: 250

- Fat: 5 grams

- Carbohydrates: 30 grams

- Fiber: 5 grams

- Protein: 15 grams

Cooking Steps	Ingredients
1. Spread the mashed tofu on the whole-wheat bread slices. 2. Add the vegetables, mustard, salt, and pepper to taste. 3. Enjoy!	- 2 slices whole-wheat bread - 1/4 cup tofu, mashed - 1/4 cup vegetables (such as tomatoes, cucumbers, or sprouts), chopped - 1 tablespoon mustard - 1/4 teaspoon salt - 1/4 teaspoon black pepper

Hard-Boiled Eggs and Whole-Wheat Crackers

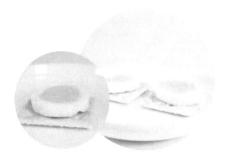

Prep time: 5 minutes

A healthy and convenient lunch choice is hard-boiled eggs and whole-wheat crackers. Hard-boiled eggs are high in protein and healthful fats. Whole-wheat crackers are high in fiber and complex carbs.

Nutritional information:

One serving of two hard-boiled eggs and six whole-wheat crackers contains approximately:

- Calories: 250

- Fat: 10 grams

- Carbohydrates: 30 grams

- Fiber: 5 grams

- Protein: 20 grams

Cooking Steps	Ingredients
Hard-boiled eggs should be peeled. Serve the hard-boiled eggs alongside whole-wheat crackers.	- 2 hard-boiled eggs - 6 whole-wheat crackers

Turkey Sandwich on Whole-Wheat Bread with Avocado and Vegetables

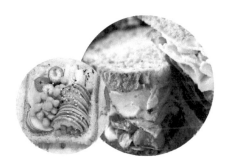

Prep time: 5 minutes

A healthy and delicious lunch option is a turkey sandwich on whole-wheat bread with avocado and vegetables. Turkey is high in protein and lean protein. Avocado is high in fiber and healthy fats. Whole-wheat bread is high in fiber and complex carbs.

Nutritional information:

One serving of a turkey sandwich on whole-wheat bread with avocado and vegetables contains approximately:

- Calories: 300

- Fat: 10 grams

- Carbohydrates: 40 grams

- Fiber: 5 grams, Protein: 20 grams

Cooking Steps	Ingredients
1. Spread the mashed avocado on the whole-wheat bread slices. 2. Add the turkey, veggies, mustard, salt, and pepper to taste. 3. Enjoy!	- 2 slices whole-wheat bread - 1/4 cup cooked turkey, sliced - 1/4 avocado, mashed - 1/4 cup vegetables (such as tomatoes, cucumbers, or sprouts), chopped - 1 tablespoon mustard - 1/4 teaspoon salt - 1/4 teaspoon black pepper

Lentil Tacos

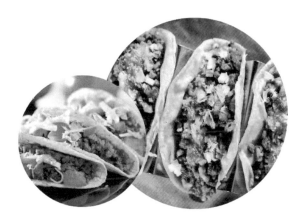

Prep time: 10 minutes _ Cook time: 10 minutes

Lentil tacos are a nutritious and tasty lunch choice. Lentils provide protein, fiber, and complex carbs. They are also low in fat and calories.

Nutritional information:

One serving of lentil tacos contains approximately:

- Calories: 250

- Fat: 5 grams

- Carbohydrates: 30 grams

- Fiber: 10 grams

- Protein: 15 grams

Cooking Steps	Ingredients
1. In a pan over medium heat, cook the lentils. 2. Cook for 5 minutes, or until the veggies are softened, with the vegetables and taco seasoning. 3. Fill taco shells with lentil mixture and top with desired toppings. 4. Enjoy!	- 1 cup lentils, cooked - 1/2 cup vegetables (such as tomatoes, onions, or peppers), chopped - 1/4 cup taco seasoning - 12 taco shells - Toppings of your choice (such as lettuce, cheese, sour cream, and guacamole)

Tips for making lentil tacos:

- Cook the lentils in vegetable broth instead of chicken stock for a vegetarian option.

- To the lentil mixture, add your favorite vegetables.

- Serve with your preferred toppings.

Variations:

- Add a dab of spicy sauce to the lentil mixture for a hotter taco.

- Use whole-wheat taco shells and low-fat cheese for a healthier taco.

- Add a side of black beans or rice for a more substantial taco.

CHAPTER SIX

TRIGLYCERIDE-LOWERING DINNER RECIPES

Grilled Salmon with Roasted Vegetables

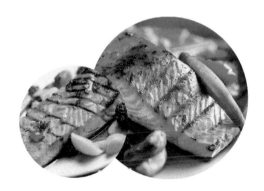

Prep time: 10 minutes _ Cook time: 20 minutes

Grilled salmon is a nutritious and tasty dinner option. Salmon is high in protein and omega-3 fatty acids. Vegetables that have been roasted are high in vitamins, minerals, and antioxidants.

Nutritional information:

One serving of grilled salmon with roasted vegetables contains approximately:

- Calories: 350

- Fat: 20 grams

- Carbohydrates: 20 grams

- Fiber: 5 grams

- Protein: 30 grams

Cooking Steps	Ingredients
1. Preheat the grill to medium-high temperature. 2. Season the salmon fillet with salt and pepper after brushing it with olive oil. 3. Grill the salmon fillet for 6-8 minutes per side, or until it is cooked through. 4. While the salmon is cooking, roast the veggies in a 400°F preheated oven for 15-20 minutes, or until soft. 5. With the roasted veggies, serve the salmon.	- 1 salmon fillet (6 ounces) - 1 tablespoon olive oil - 1/4 teaspoon salt - 1/4 teaspoon black pepper - 1 cup vegetables (such as broccoli, Brussels sprouts, or sweet potatoes), chopped

Chicken Stir-Fry with Brown Rice

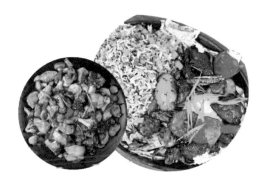

Prep time: 10 minutes _ Cook time: 15 minutes

Chicken stir-fry is a nutritious and tasty dinner alternative. Stir-fries are a quick and simple way to prepare veggies and meats. Brown rice is high in complex carbs and fiber.

Nutritional information:

One serving of chicken stir-fry with brown rice contains approximately:

- Calories: 350

- Fat: 10 grams

- Carbohydrates: 40 grams

- Fiber: 5 grams

- Protein: 30 grams

Cooking Steps	Ingredients
1. In a large skillet over medium-high heat, heat the olive oil. 2. Cook for 5-7 minutes, or until the chicken is cooked through, in the skillet. 3. Stir in the soy sauce, ginger powder, garlic powder, and black pepper to mix. 4. Cook for 3-5 minutes, or until the vegetables are soft, in the skillet. 5. Serve the stir-fry chicken over brown rice.	- 1 pound chicken breast, cut into bite-sized pieces - 1 tablespoon olive oil - 1 tablespoon soy sauce - 1 teaspoon ginger powder - 1/2 teaspoon garlic powder - 1/4 teaspoon black pepper - 1 cup vegetables (such as broccoli, carrots, or bell peppers), chopped - 1 cup cooked brown rice

Tofu Tacos with Quinoa and Vegetables

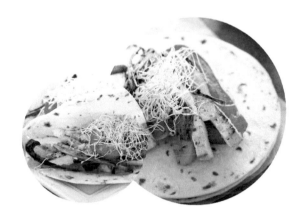

Prep time: 10 minutes _ Cook time: 15 minutes

Tofu tacos are a nutritious and tasty dinner choice. Tacos are a tasty and convenient way to consume vegetables and protein. Quinoa has both protein and fiber.

Nutritional information:

One serving of tofu tacos with quinoa and vegetables contains approximately:

- Calories: 350

- Fat: 10 grams

- Carbohydrates: 40 grams

- Fiber: 10 grams

- Protein: 30 grams

Cooking Steps	Ingredients
1. In a large skillet over medium heat, heat the olive oil. 2. Cook the tofu in the skillet for 5-7 minutes, or until browned. 3. Cook for 3-5 minutes, or until the veggies are cooked, in the skillet with the vegetables and taco seasoning. 4. Fill taco shells with tofu mixture and top with desired toppings. 5. Tacos should be served with quinoa.	- 1 block tofu, crumbled - 1 tablespoon olive oil - 1/2 cup vegetables (such as tomatoes, onions, or peppers), chopped - 1/4 cup taco seasoning - 12 taco shells - Toppings of your choice (such as lettuce, cheese, sour cream, and guacamole) - 1 cup cooked quinoa

Spaghetti with Whole-Wheat Pasta and Tomato Sauce

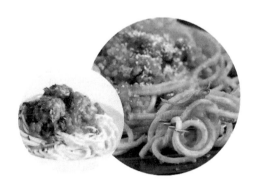

Prep time: 10 minutes _ Cook time: 20 minutes

A healthy and delicious dinner choice is spaghetti with whole-wheat noodles and tomato sauce. Whole-wheat pasta is high in fiber and complex carbs. Tomato sauce contains vitamins, minerals, and antioxidants.

Nutritional information:

One serving of spaghetti with whole-wheat pasta and tomato sauce contains approximately:

- Calories: 500
- Fat: 10 grams
- Carbohydrates: 70 grams
- Fiber: 10 grams

- Protein: 20 grams

Cooking Steps	Ingredients
1. Cook the spaghetti as directed on the packet. 2. In a large saucepan over medium heat, heat the olive oil while the spaghetti is cooking. 3. Cook for 5 minutes, or until the onion and garlic are softened, in the pot. 4. Bring the crushed tomatoes, oregano, basil, salt, and pepper to a simmer in a saucepan. 5. Reduce the heat to low and continue to cook for 15 minutes, or until the sauce has thickened. 6. Return the pasta to the pot after draining. 7. Toss the spaghetti with the tomato sauce and Parmesan cheese to incorporate. 8. Serve right away.	- 1 pound whole-wheat spaghetti - 1 (28-ounce) can of whole peeled tomatoes, crushed by hand - 1/2 onion, chopped - 2 cloves garlic, minced - 1/4 teaspoon dried oregano - 1/4 teaspoon dried basil - 1/4 teaspoon salt - 1/4 teaspoon black pepper - 1/4 cup grated Parmesan cheese

Tips for making spaghetti with whole-wheat pasta and tomato sauce:

- To lower the sodium content of the recipe, use low-sodium canned tomatoes.

- To the tomato sauce, add your favorite vegetables, such as mushrooms, zucchini, or spinach.

- For a complete supper, serve with a side salad or grilled chicken.

Black Bean Burgers with Sweet Potato Fries

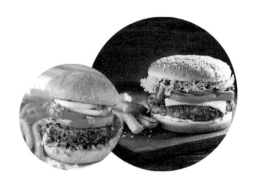

Prep time: 20 minutes _ Cook time: 30 minutes

Black bean burgers are a nutritious and tasty dinner alternative. Black beans are high in protein and fiber. Vitamins, minerals, and antioxidants are abundant in sweet potato fries.

Nutritional information:

One serving of black bean burgers with sweet potato fries contains approximately:

- Calories: 600
- Fat: 20 grams
- Carbohydrates: 70 grams
- Fiber: 10 grams
- Protein: 20 grams

Cooking Steps	Ingredients
1. Preheat the oven to 400° Fahrenheit.	- 1 (15-ounce) can black beans, rinsed and drained
2. Combine the black beans, onion, brown rice, breadcrumbs, egg, chili powder, cumin, salt, and pepper in a large mixing bowl.	- 1/2 onion, chopped - 1/2 cup cooked brown rice
3. Form the mixture into four patties.	- 1/4 cup breadcrumbs - 1 egg, beaten
4. In a large skillet over medium heat, heat the vegetable oil.	- 1 tablespoon chili powder
5. Cook for 5-7 minutes per side, or until the burgers are browned and cooked through.	- 1 teaspoon cumin - 1/4 teaspoon salt
6. Bake the sweet potato fries according to package directions while the burgers are cooking.	- 1/4 teaspoon black pepper
7. With the sweet potato fries, serve the burgers.	- 1/4 cup vegetable oil - 1 (16-ounce) package of sweet potato fries

Tips for making black bean burgers with sweet potato fries:

- Top the burgers with your favorite toppings, such as cheese, lettuce, tomato, and avocado.

- Serve with a dipping sauce of your choice, such as ketchup, mustard, or salsa.

- Cook the burgers in a nonstick skillet for a healthier choice.

Grilled Chicken Breast with Brown Rice and Vegetables

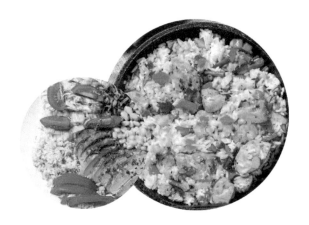

Nutritional information:

One serving of grilled chicken breast with brown rice and vegetables contains approximately:

- Calories: 350

- Fat: 10 grams

- Carbohydrates: 40 grams

- Fiber: 5 grams

- Protein: 30 grams

Cooking Steps	Ingredients
1. Preheat the grill to medium-high temperature. 2. Season the chicken breast with salt and pepper after brushing it with olive oil. 3. Cook the chicken breast for 6-8 minutes per side on the grill, or until cooked through. 4. With brown rice and roasted veggies, serve the chicken breast.	- 1 boneless, skinless chicken breast (6 ounces) - 1 tablespoon olive oil - 1/4 teaspoon salt - 1/4 teaspoon black pepper - 1 cup brown rice, cooked - 1 cup vegetables (such as broccoli, Brussels sprouts, or sweet potatoes), roasted

Vegetarian Chili

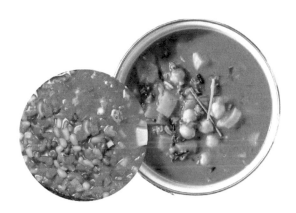

Nutritional information:

One serving of vegetarian chili contains approximately:

- Calories: 250
- Fat: 5 grams
- Carbohydrates: 40 grams
- Fiber: 10 grams
- Protein: 15 grams

Cooking Steps	Ingredients
1. In a large pot over medium heat, heat the olive oil.	- 1 tablespoon olive oil
2. Cook for 5 minutes, or until the onion, garlic, and bell pepper are softened.	- 1 onion, chopped - 2 cloves garlic, minced - 1 green bell pepper, chopped
3. To the pot, include the kidney beans, black beans, diced tomatoes, corn, vegetable broth, chili powder, cumin, salt, and pepper.	- 2 (15-ounce) cans of kidney beans, rinsed and drained - 2 (15-ounce) cans of black beans, rinsed and drained - 1 (14.5-ounce) can of diced tomatoes, undrained
4. Bring the chili to a boil, then reduce to low heat and continue to cook for 15 minutes, or until the chili has thickened.	- 1 (10-ounce) can of corn kernels, drained - 1 (10-ounce) can vegetable broth - 1 teaspoon chili powder
5. Serve the chili immediately.	- 1/2 teaspoon cumin - 1/4 teaspoon salt - 1/4 teaspoon black pepper

Salmon with Roasted Vegetables

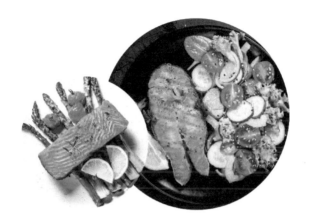

Nutritional information:

One serving of salmon with roasted vegetables contains approximately:

- Calories: 350

- Fat: 20 grams

- Carbohydrates: 20 grams

- Fiber: 5 grams

- Protein: 30 grams

Cooking Steps	Ingredients
1. Preheat the oven to 400° Fahrenheit.	- 1 (6-ounce) salmon fillet
2. Season the salmon fillet with salt and pepper after brushing it with olive oil.	- 1 tablespoon olive oil - 1/4 teaspoon salt
3. Cook the salmon fillet for 12-15 minutes, or until cooked through, on a baking pan.	- 1/4 teaspoon black pepper
4. With roasted vegetables, serve the salmon.	- 1 cup vegetables (such as broccoli, Brussels sprouts, or sweet potatoes), roasted

.

CHAPTER SEVEN

TRIGLYCERIDE-LOWERING

SNACKS RECIPES

Fruits and Vegetables

Fruits and vegetables are a healthy and delicious snack option. They are a good source of vitamins, minerals, and antioxidants. They are also low in calories and fat.

Cooking Steps	Ingredients
1. Wash and chop the fruits and vegetables. 2. Enjoy! 3. Prep time: 5 minutes	1 cup of fruits and vegetables of your choice (such as berries, bananas, carrots, or celery)

Nutritional information:

One serving of fruits and vegetables contains approximately:

- Calories: 50
- Fat: 0 grams
- Carbohydrates: 15 grams
- Fiber: 5 grams
- Protein: 0 grams

Nuts and Seeds

Nuts and seeds are a healthy and satisfying snack option. They are a good source of protein, fiber, and healthy fats. They can also be a good source of vitamins and minerals, depending on the type of nut or seed.

Cooking Steps	Ingredients
1. Prep time: 5 minutes 2. Enjoy!	1/4 cup nuts and seeds of your choice (such as almonds, walnuts, chia seeds, or flaxseeds)

Nutritional information:

One serving of nuts and seeds contains approximately:

- Calories: 150
- Fat: 10 grams
- Carbohydrates: 5 grams
- Fiber: 3 grams
- Protein: 5 grams

Yogurt

Yogurt is a healthy and delicious snack option. It is a good source of protein, calcium, and other nutrients. It can also be a good source of probiotics, which are beneficial bacteria that can help improve gut health.

Cooking Steps	Ingredients
1. Prep time: 5 minutes 2. Enjoy!	1 cup yogurt of your choice

Nutritional information:

One serving of yogurt contains approximately:

- Calories: 100
- Fat: 0 grams
- Carbohydrates: 15 grams
- Fiber: 0 grams
- Protein: 10 grams

Hard-Boiled Eggs

Hard-boiled eggs are a healthy and convenient snack option. They are a good source of protein and healthy fats. They are also low in calories.

Cooking Steps	Ingredients
1. Prep time: 5 minutes 2. Peel the hard-boiled egg. 3. Enjoy!	1 hard-boiled egg

Nutritional information:

One hard-boiled egg contains approximately:

- Calories: 75
- Fat: 5 grams
- Carbohydrates: 1 gram
- Fiber: 0 grams
- Protein: 6 grams

Whole-Wheat Crackers

Whole-wheat crackers are a healthy and satisfying snack option. They are a good source of complex carbohydrates and fiber. They can also be a good source of vitamins and minerals, depending on the type of cracker.

Cooking Steps	Ingredients
Prep time: 5 minutes Enjoy!	6 whole-wheat crackers

Nutritional information:

Six whole-wheat crackers contain approximately:

- Calories: 100
- Fat: 2 grams
- Carbohydrates: 20 grams
- Fiber: 3 grams
- Protein: 3 grams

Trail Mix

Trail mix is a healthy and convenient snack option. It is a good source of protein, fiber, and healthy fats. It can also be a good source of vitamins and minerals, depending on the ingredients in the trail mix.

Cooking Steps	Ingredients
Prep time: 5 minutes Enjoy!	1/4 cup trail mix (made with nuts, seeds, and dried fruit)

Nutritional information:

1/4 cup of trail mix contains approximately:

- Calories: 150
- Fat: 10 grams
- Carbohydrates: 10 grams
- Fiber: 3 grams
- Protein: 5 grams

Edamame

Edamame is a healthy and delicious snack option. It is a good source of protein, fiber, and antioxidants. It is also low in calories and fat.

Cooking Steps	Ingredients
1. Cook the edamame according to package directions. 2. Let the edamame cool slightly. 3. Enjoy! 4. Prep time: 5 minutes	1 cup edamame

Nutritional information:

One cup of edamame contains approximately:

- Calories: 150
- Fat: 5 grams
- Carbohydrates: 20 grams
- Fiber: 5 grams
- Protein: 10 grams

Hard Cheese and Whole-Wheat Crackers

Hard cheese and whole-wheat crackers are a healthy and satisfying snack option. Hard cheese is a good source of protein, calcium, and other nutrients. Whole-wheat crackers are a good source of complex carbohydrates and fiber.

Cooking Steps	Ingredients
1. Cut the cheese into cubes.	- 1 ounce hard cheese
2. Enjoy the cheese with the whole-wheat crackers.	- 6 whole-wheat crackers
3. Prep time: 5 minutes	

Nutritional information:

One ounce of hard cheese and six whole-wheat crackers contain approximately:

- Calories: 200
- Fat: 10 grams
- Carbohydrates: 25 grams
- Fiber: 5 grams, Protein: 10 grams

Hummus with Whole-Wheat Pita Bread

Hummus is a healthy and delicious snack option. It is a good source of protein, fiber, and healthy fats. Whole-wheat pita bread is a good source of complex carbohydrates and fiber.

Cooking Steps	Ingredients
1. Cut the pita bread into triangles.	- 1/4 cup hummus
2. Spread the hummus on the pita bread triangles.	- 1 whole-wheat pita bread
3. Enjoy!	
4. Prep time: 5 minutes	

Nutritional information:

1/4 cup of hummus and one whole-wheat pita bread contain approximately: Calories: 250

- Fat: 10 grams
- Carbohydrates: 30 grams
- Fiber: 5 grams
- Protein: 10 grams

Smoothie Made with Fruits, Vegetables, and Yogurt

Smoothies are a healthy and delicious snack option. They are a good way to get your daily dose of fruits and vegetables. They can also be a good source of protein and fiber, depending on the ingredients in the smoothie.

Cooking Steps	Ingredients
1. Combine all of the ingredients in a blender and blend until smooth. 2. Enjoy! 3. Prep time: 5 minutes	- 1 cup yogurt - 1/2 cup fruit (such as berries, banana, or mango) - 1/2 cup vegetables (such as spinach, kale, or cucumber) - 1/2 cup water or milk

Nutritional information:

One serving of smoothie made with fruits, vegetables, and yogurt contains approximately:

- Calories: 250
- Fat: 5 grams
- Carbohydrates: 40 grams
- Fiber: 10 grams
- Protein: 10 grams

Conclusion

Lowering triglycerides is an important element of keeping your heart healthy and lowering your risk of heart disease and other chronic health problems. By making the dietary and lifestyle modifications recommended in this book, you can improve your triglyceride levels as well as your general health and well-being.

The following are some major insights from this book:

- Consume a diet reduced in saturated and trans fats, sweets, and sodium.
- Exercise regularly. On most days of the week, aim for at least 30 minutes of moderate-intensity exercise.
- If you are overweight or obese, you should lose weight. Even minor weight loss might have a significant impact on your triglyceride levels.

Consult your doctor if you have any questions or concerns regarding your triglyceride levels. They can assist you in developing a tailored plan to reduce your triglycerides and enhance your overall health.

Remember that your health is your most valuable asset. You can live a longer, healthier, and happier life if you take care of yourself.

Manufactured by Amazon.ca
Bolton, ON